I0102145

A DAY
IN THE LIFE OF A
PHLEBOTOMIST

Outpatient Laboratory *Edition*

Jonathan I. Angulo

Legal Notice

Disclaimer

This is a book of non-fiction and the stories told here are true, collected from the time I worked as a phlebotomist in an outpatient laboratory. Events in the book are reproduced to the best of my memory, though I have altered some details for clarity. Other details have been modified to conceal the identities of patients and coworkers, and in the interest of protecting patients' and coworkers' confidentiality.

A DAY
IN THE LIFE OF A
PHLEBOTOMIST

Outpatient Laboratory *Edition*

Contents

A DAY
IN THE LIFE OF A
PHLEBOTOMIST
with ε Outpatient Laboratory Edition

Chapter One

A Bright New Day

As the clock turns to 7:00 a.m., I know it's time to get going. I zip up my hoodie and grab my lunch, all while trying not to make a lot of noise since my family is still asleep, and with that I am ready to leave my house. Leaving any later will not give me enough time should there be an accident or more traffic than usual on our already congested Los Angeles freeways. Fortunately, it is February and the days are starting to get bright earlier, and that usually makes traffic a little better in the mornings because drivers are able to see better.

As I make my way to the car, I'm hoping that I can get to work with some time to spare, especially since today is Monday, the busiest day of the week at the laboratory, and I'm the only phlebotomist there. I'm also the one who opens up the gates and lets the patients into the building. So, getting there late would probably mean getting the attitude of hungry patients who have been fasting—not consuming any food or liquids other than water—since last night. Some patients have been waiting outside in the cold for an hour or more because they want to be the first one I help out, just so they can get it over with and enjoy the rest of their day. That's why I always try to be there as early as possible—to avoid any more suffering for them, and for me as well.

I get in my car and begin driving, and soon enough I am joining the freeway in my old 2002 Mustang GT. I roll down the windows to get that morning chilly wind in my face—it always works wonders on Mondays to make me more alert as I drive half-asleep. The sight of a nicely flowing freeway makes me happy, because that means I will have enough time to stop by the McDonald's near my workplace and pick up a coffee to warm me up this cold morning and help me start the day.

McDonald's holds a very special place in my heart because it's where I worked to pay my tuition when I went to phlebotomy school last year. Although a lot of people complain about working there, I always saw the good of it. A steady job, lots of hours available, flexible schedule, and the opportunity to grow within the company. But what I miss the most is the conversations and relationships that I was able to build with some of my coworkers.

I still remember working a shift there as manager when I got a call from the supervisor at the laboratory. I had met the supervisor during my clinical internship at the lab when I was training to become a phlebotomist—a medical professional who draws blood and takes other samples from patients. The supervisor was at the laboratory almost daily because the place was about to change ownership and she had to help with the transitioning. I suppose me being a team player while I was learning there left a great impression on her, which was why she decided to call me for a job interview. The previous phlebotomist, who taught me during my internship, had moved away, and the supervisor thought I could be a good fit since I already knew how the business operated.

Sometimes it still feels surreal that I was able to get this job at such a young age. I still wonder if it was pure luck or my actual qualities. How could I, a 20-year-old, be running that place almost by myself? How did I transition so quickly from being an inexperienced student phlebotomist at this exact same place to being the only phlebotomist in charge of opening, closing, and helping patients of all ages?

While the answer is still unknown to me, I want to believe that it was a little bit of both luck and hard work that got me here. Regardless of the reason, I committed to work in healthcare in order to do good for people, and this job is allowing me to do just that.

After a 12-mile drive through the local freeways and streets, here I am at the McDonald's drive-thru at 7:40 a.m., about a mile from the lab, waiting to get my coffee. While I wait, I begin creating a mental checklist of the things I will have to do once I get to work and before opening the door for patients to come inside the lab. This way, I will already know what to do when I get there and will not waste any time.

As I am driving past the building before I park, the smell of coffee hanging in the air in my car, I get a glance at the people standing outside waiting for me to open the gates. Since the lab is inside a square-shaped single-floor building surrounded by other medical offices, all of the patients have to wait outside for me to open the gates and allow them inside, regardless of which office they are visiting. Today there are about 15 people standing outside already. Oh, god, it seems like it's going to be one of those busy Mondays. Good thing I had time to grab coffee, because I am going to need the caffeine boost. I park my car, take a deep breath, and here I go to help out patients to the best of my ability.

Chapter Two

8:00 a.m

As I walk toward the crowd, I note that the majority of them are elderly patients wearing sweaters or vests. Some of them wear sombreros, and two of them are also carrying canes. As I get closer, some of them are already looking at me with piercing eyes. Although it is still 15 minutes away from the time I open our lab doors, and I am technically early to open the gates, to our hungry and elderly patients, I'm late already. They surely wish I was here 30 minutes ago, just so they could come inside and shelter from the cold while sitting down.

I totally understand why they get upset, and as a matter of fact some patients might not have control over their anger or anxiety. The reason is because some elderly patients—and the majority of patients who get here this early are elderly—have diabetes, and some of them have not had anything to eat or drink in the past 12 hours. This might cause their blood sugar levels to go slightly down, and when that happens they can become anxious and upset. Combine that with some patients who might tend to be cranky by nature, and you get a bad combination.

I get to the gates and say "good morning" to everyone, and the patients say good morning back to me. I unlock the gates and allow them in before me. One of them stays behind while the rest rush inside and make a line outside the lab doors. This happens every single time. The patient who stayed behind asks me for directions to one of the eight doctor's offices in the building, and I direct him to the right place. I walk around the lab and enter it through our employees-only side door. Here I go: once I cross this door, I will be committed to being in here for the next nine hours. What I would give to be at a beach with nicer weather enjoying a fresh cold drink, but for now I've got to take care of all of these patients.

The moment I get inside, I feel a sense of urgency. The clock is ticking . . . tick-tock! I recall the mental checklist I made for myself earlier and start working on it. I turn on all of the inside lights with exception of the light in the waiting room, because once the patients see that light from outside they immediately begin trying to open the door to come in. Next, I put out a new sign-in sheet on the clipboard and put paper in the copier machine. I use the copier a lot—I need to copy every single patient's laboratory order, or lab order for short, for our billing and records. Last but not least, I give the floor a quick sweep and check the restroom to make sure there is toilet paper. You can never underestimate the importance of having enough toilet paper!

Once I make sure that the place looks neat and is ready to welcome patients, I check my actual working area inside the lab. I look at my watch, and I still have five minutes left before I let the first patient in. I log into the computer and open the websites to the outside laboratories that we are contracted with. Each of these websites has a test menu where I can look up any test that was ordered by the doctor and learn vital information about the test, such as if there are any special instructions to collect it, how much blood to collect, what color tube it needs to be collected in. I also put on a playlist of relaxing music to create a nice, calm environment for the patients, since some of them are really afraid of having their blood drawn. A soft piano melody drifts over the room.

Next, I make sure I have enough of the most common empty tubes to collect blood immediately in my working area. This way I don't have to be looking for them once I call in the patients. I also check that I have enough supply of needles, vacutainer hubs, cotton balls, alcohol swabs, bandages, lollipops for children, and tourniquets—the elastic disposable rubber bands that I tie around patients' arms to help make the veins pop out.

Lastly, I check the puncture-proof sharps container where I discard of used needles. It's almost full, so I pull a new sharps container out of the utility room, attach the non-removable lid to it, and place it nearby to swap them when the old one becomes full.

Now I'm ready to begin the day, fully stocked and ready for whatever comes my way. Or almost ready—I have a few more sips of my coffee left, so I sit down and enjoy it for these last two minutes.

Finally the time has come: it is 8:00 a.m. I turn on the lights in the waiting room and unlock and open the front door, and patients begin coming in. I rush inside, get behind the desk, and begin seeing the patients as they write down their names and hand me their lab orders one by one through the reception window. My interaction with each patient is almost the same: I smile, grab their order and, depending on the tests, I ask them, "Are you fasting today?" If they say yes, I tell them, "Okay, perfect, have a seat please." Most patients who are supposed to be fasting do show up that way, but occasionally I get patients who have had something to eat or drink already.

Today is no different. Everyone answers yes except for one patient. He is a man who looks to be in his 60s or 70s, wearing a sombrero and carrying an old-fashioned cane carved out of wood.

"Nobody told me to be fasting, I already drank my coffee and sweet bread," he says in Spanish, his voice rising. He is starting to realize that his trip to the lab may have been a waste of time. "Can't we just do it anyway?"

"I'm sorry," I tell him in Spanish. "For these tests, your doctor wants you to be fasting, so I can't draw your blood today. It would interfere with the results, and you don't want that, right? You'll have to come back tomorrow fasting, and I'll be glad to help you out."

He stands there staring at me for an extra few seconds, just to let me know how mad he is, but it's not my fault! I have to make sure that every patient who is supposed to be fasting is indeed fasting. Luckily, this patient turns away with a grumble and heads out the door. Some patients get really upset that I'm turning them back after they wasted their morning and waited outside in the cold, but doing those tests if they haven't been fasting could severely alter their test's results, and that is not a good thing for them.

The other thing I have to do for each patient is make sure their lab order is from an outside laboratory that we are contracted with. As an outpatient laboratory, we draw blood and take other samples from patients, but we send these samples to an outside laboratory to be tested. If a patient's lab order is not from one of the contracted outside labs, that is another reason why I might have to turn them away. Sadly, since we are an outpatient laboratory, people sometimes come with lab orders from other labs and expect us to do their tests. However, if we are not contracted with that outside laboratory, we do not get reimbursement from them, and that particular lab might not come and pick up the specimens even if we do draw their blood, thus the patient will have had their blood drawn for no reason.

Today, everyone's lab order is from a contracted lab, so once every patient has signed in and had their questions answered, I put all of their lab orders in the right order, put the first one in the front, and place them all on a wall-mounted file holder I have outside of the draw station where I draw the blood. New lab orders will go in the back as more patients arrive. As for now, it is showtime—time to begin taking care of the patients.

Chapter Three

Showtime

I grab the first lab order and take it to my draw station—a table built against the wall in a corner with a cabinet on top that I use to keep some supplies. Here, I quickly take a look at it and make sure that the lab order has the minimum information I need to be able to help the patient. The first thing I check is whether all the administrative parts are taken care of.

The lab order must have the patient's name and date of birth at the very minimum. It also needs to have the diagnosis code(s). All diseases or injuries in America and other countries are assigned a diagnosis code called an ICD (International Classification of Diseases) for standardization and easy identification across medical and insurance personnel. Some orders may also include the patient's address and other information, but that is not important for me to perform my job.

While at school we are taught that in order to identify a patient accurately, we must have at least two unique patient identifiers. Correctly identifying a patient is so important to avoid putting patients at risk. Imagine patient A, who has the same name as patient B, getting lab results showing that he has a disease he in fact does not have. That would make patient A get treated for something he doesn't have, while patient B is not getting the treatment he might need to save his life. That is why a patient's name and a date of birth are so important to have on the lab order. I use those two to identify the patients once I call them back. I also handwrite those two identifiers on all specimens collected from each patient, be it tubes filled with blood or urine containers.

Insurance information is not needed for me to proceed with the draw, but it is needed for billing purposes. Without it, the outside laboratory that will test the patient's samples might not get reimbursed from the patient's insurance, and that would result in the patient getting billed for the tests.

If any of these important details are missing from a lab order, I might be able to resolve it by calling the patient's doctor's office and asking for the missing information. For example, I can usually get the diagnosis code or insurance information from the doctor's office. I can sometimes get insurance information from the patient themself. If the missing part is the name or date of birth, due to our own policies, I need to send the patient away.

For my first patient today, the lab order reads: Maria Hernandez, 5/5/1956. ICD codes are there, but the insurance information is missing. I make a mental note of this for myself. Since Mrs. Hernandez's lab order has the minimum information I need in order to securely identify who she is, I can read the rest of the lab order and identify what tests were ordered for the patient. For Mrs. Hernandez, the tests ordered are: CMP, LP, CBC, HgbA1c, and UA complete. Those names are actually the tests abbreviated, which makes it easier for us to work with them. For example, CMP stands for Comprehensive Metabolic Panel, and LP stands for Lipid Panel. It's way easier for us to just say CMP or LP.

The tests Mrs. Hernandez's doctor has ordered are routine labs. She is having blood drawn and urine collected to check how well her kidneys and liver are working. She is also having her electrolytes checked. The doctor also requested to test for her cholesterol levels, a test to check if she's diabetic, and another one to see if she's anemic. Due to the tests ordered for her, she needs to be fasting today.

I really like when patients come with lab orders with common tests ordered, at least during the busy times in the morning. This helps me get to patients sooner because I do not have to do any research on how to collect those specimens or make sure there are no special requirements for the test ordered. For example, sometimes I need to collect the sample only during the morning, or perhaps I need to protect it from light by wrapping the tube in foil paper. Other times the sample must be collected without applying a tourniquet, and sometimes I need to put the specimen in the refrigerator right away.

I go to the cabinet and grab one tiger-top tube and one lavender tube. We call the tubes by the colors of the top stopper. Depending on the tests ordered, more than one test can be conducted on the same test tube. In this case, CMP and LP will both be tested out of the tiger-top; CBC and HgbA1c will be tested out of the lavender tube.

I also grab an alcohol pad, a cotton ball, bandage, tourniquet, urine cup, needle, and vacutainer hub. The vacutainer hub is a small transparent plastic device that attaches to the needle and helps connect the needle to the plastic tube safely. The entire process of getting ready to call the patient from the time I pick up their lab order usually takes me about three minutes.

I walk over to the reception area, open the waiting room door, and call out, "Maria Hernandez." I then see a nicely dressed lady stand up and walk towards me. "Good morning, this way please, have a seat on that chair," I say as I point towards the chair adjacent to the draw station table.

She smiles back at me, has a seat, and instantly rolls up the sleeve of her left arm and rests it on the table. As soon as she does, I notice that she has a nice vein that I can work with. I will just need to feel it to make sure, but for now it looks like it will be a good one.

At this point, I once more need to verify her identity: "Mrs. Hernandez, can you please tell me your full name and your date of birth?"

She answers, "Maria Hernandez, 5/5/1956."

Perfect. I then say, "Mrs. Hernandez, I see no insurance information on your lab order, and I don't want you to end up getting a bill from the laboratory. May I borrow your insurance card for a minute?"

She hands me her insurance card, and I quickly make a copy of it and staple it to her lab order. It's not mandatory for me to verify billing information, but some patients are already sick and going through a lot in their lives, and I feel that the least I can do is try to help them avoid the stress of hefty bills from the laboratories. After all, that is why we are here, to help out the patients and not cause them any more headaches.

Next, I need to make sure that she is actually fasting, and that she understands what fasting actually means, as some patients surprisingly do not know. So, I ask her, "When was the last time you ate or had anything to drink other than water?"

"Last night before bed, around 9:00 p.m.," she responds.

Everything checks out then. "We will be needing bloodwork and a urine sample as well today, okay, Mrs. Hernandez?"

"No problem" she responds.

I put gloves on, tie the tourniquet around her arm, and palpate or feel for the previously eyeballed vein in her antecubital fossa—the area at the bend of the arm, opposite to the elbow. It's difficult to explain how to identify a good vein, but in a nutshell, we feel for a bouncy feeling of the vein once we push on it with our fingers. Also, a vein has a different feeling from other human tissues. At some point, it became second nature for me to begin looking at patients' arms in search of a usable vein even without thinking about doing it. Thankfully, Mrs. Hernandez's vein looks and feels like one that I can easily use to draw her blood.

I open the alcohol pad and, as I rub it on Mrs. Hernandez's arm to clean the area where I'm going to draw the blood, a whiff of alcohol fills the air. Cleaning the area before drawing blood is important because it helps ensure that we are not introducing any germs to the patient's circulation as we draw their blood. Alcohol does the trick because it kills the germs. While the alcohol on her arm dries, I screw the needle and the vacutainer hub together and open the packaging of the bandage.

Now I remove the cap from the needle and rest my hand, which is holding the needle, on her arm. Doing this helps me keep my hand steady while drawing her blood, which is particularly important because any unnecessary movement of my hand could cause her some pain if the needle moves back and forth while inside of her arm.

At the same time that I'm resting my right hand on her arm, I use my left thumb to pull down on her skin about three inches below where I will poke her with the needle. This helps me make sure that her vein doesn't move so I don't miss and have to poke her again.

With a swift motion, I pierce her skin with the needle. Once I do so, I release the skin I was pulling with my left hand and use that hand to grab a tiger-top tube. As soon as it begins to fill up with blood, I remove the tourniquet. It's important not to leave the tourniquet on for more than one to two minutes at a time, because doing so might cause some tests to be inaccurate. Once the tiger-top tube is full, I remove it from inside the vacutainer hub and insert the lavender tube.

The order in which we select the tubes to fill up with blood is not random. We have what we call "the order of draw," which is a predetermined order that might vary from laboratory to laboratory depending on the equipment they use to test the blood. The order of draw is important because almost all tubes have some chemicals inside of them to help preserve the blood, and not all chemicals are compatible with other chemicals, so we need to avoid the chemicals coming in contact with each other as we switch from one tube to another. If two incompatible chemicals mix with each other, some of those tubes might not be able to get tested at the laboratory, or the results might come out inaccurate.

Now that the lavender tube is full of blood, I remove it from the vacutainer hub, grab the cotton ball next to me with my left hand, and place it on Mrs. Hernandez's arm where the needle is. Then I swiftly remove the needle from her arm and engage the safety lock that the needle has attached to it to prevent from accidental punctures. Then I dispose of it in the sharps container next to me. I gently invert the two tubes a few times to make sure the blood mixes evenly with the chemicals inside of them. Lastly, I put the bandage on top of the cotton ball on her arm.

Now that I've finished drawing her blood, I immediately label the tubes with Mrs. Hernandez's information. I write down her full name, her date of birth, and the date and time I drew her blood. Then I do the same thing with a urine cup and hand it to her.

"Mrs. Hernandez, here is a cup for you to collect some urine," I tell her. "The restroom is down the hall, third door to your right. Once you're done, please bring it back here and place it on this plate. After that, you are free to go. Your doctor will receive your lab results in about one week." She grabs the cup, nods in understanding, and off she goes.

Yes! That was an easy draw. I put her tubes in a tubes holder next to the plate for the urine cups. I write my initials and the time I collected her blood on the lab order, make a photocopy of it for our records and billing, and grab the next patient's lab order.

I glance at the lab order, make sure everything is in order about it, gather my supplies, and call in the next patient. While I'm drawing this patient's blood, I hear someone come into the waiting room and call out, "Hello, anyone here?"

I yell back while having the needle inside the patient's arm, "Yes, I will be right there, please sign in your name and have a seat."

Shortly after, Mrs. Hernandez comes back from the restroom and asks, "Where do I put this?"

I sigh in my mind because this happens almost every time. It doesn't matter how specific I am when giving patients instructions about where to put their urine cup in hopes that they will not interrupt me while I am helping another patient. They just come back and ask again as if I never explained to them. I respond, "Right here, Mrs. Hernandez, on this plate please."

The same process continues for the next few patients. I look at my watch, and it is 9:00 a.m. already. Where in the world is Deborah, the receptionist? Is she going to be late on a Monday, really? The busiest day of the week, come on. As I am about to call in the next patient, I hear the employees-only door open. Woo-hoo! I say in my mind as Deborah comes in with a smile on her face and carrying two coffee cups. Suddenly my day becomes a little better as she hands me one of the coffees and takes her place in the reception area. Nothing better than that first sip of a brand-new coffee to get me pumped up for many more patients to come.

Chapter Four

A Challenging Time

Deborah is sincerely such a nice and calm person. She began working here shortly after I was hired, and her job is to take care of the reception area while I focus on patient care. She is sometimes late to work, but thankfully she always makes up for it by helping me in the lab even though that's not really part of her job.

I look at my watch and it is now 10:05 a.m. I have helped 10 patients, and so far they have all been easy draws, which means it was easy to draw their blood and there was no need for multiple attempts. I could not be happier about that. Having a difficult draw could be catastrophic, especially if it happens to be one of the early patients, because they require a lot of time. Time is of the essence during the early hours of the day, since I have a waiting room full of hungry patients wanting to go home as soon as possible. Did I mention that already? I'm sure I did. I'm not being repetitive for no reason, that's just how important is to help out those patients as soon as possible—for everyone's sake.

I take the last sip of the coffee Deborah brought me and grab the next lab order. "You have to be kidding me," I say in a very low voice that only I can hear. About 15 different tests have been ordered for this patient. I recognize the names of the tests, and I instantly know that they are for patients who have or are suspected of having Lupus—an inflammatory disease in which the patient's own immune system attacks itself.

The downside about these tests is that they are not often ordered, and the samples need some additional processing after or before I collect them. I sometimes think of tests that are not common or that have a name I cannot even pronounce as "weird tests." Those weird tests often require me to go to the particular outside laboratory's test menu on the computer and look at their instructions on how to collect and handle that specimen, and that's what I'm about to do for this patient.

I make my way to the computer, open the appropriate test menu, and begin doing my research. I sigh at the thought of how much work this particular patient is going to be and how far behind it could potentially push me, meaning the poor other patients will have to wait longer. I think I just jinxed myself by thinking about the day going very well so far, but I did not even say it out loud. Isn't jinxing only supposed to happen if I say it out loud or to someone else? Anyway, what's done is done, and now I have to push through and get to it.

I look at the first test, called Antinuclear Antibodies, or ANA for short, and type it exactly as it's displayed on the lab order. The website tells me that for this test, I need to draw one tiger-top tube, and once it has been drawn and spun in the centrifuge, I need to separate the serum with a pipette and transfer that serum to another tube that has no chemicals in it. Serum is the liquid that remains in the top part of some tubes, like the tiger-top tube, after the blood has clotted and has been spun in a centrifuge machine, which is the device that separates blood components by spinning at high speeds. After that, I need to place that tube with the serum in the refrigerator because that test needs to be refrigerated to maintain its stability until it reaches the outside laboratory that will do the testing on it.

In this way, I look up all the tests and learn the specific instructions that each one requires. It takes me about 10 to 15 minutes. I just hope this patient has some good veins and it's not a difficult draw.

Due to how surprised I was at seeing so many tests ordered for this patient, I almost forgot to verify the details of the lab order, so I do that now. Name: Elizabeth Campos, 12/01/1952. ICD codes are present, and the insurance information is also there—sweet! Everything checks out. Before calling her in, I gather my supplies, which includes ten tubes in total. Ten tubes! This is going to take me a little bit.

I walk over to the reception area and take a quick glance at what Deborah is doing on the computer as I open the waiting room door. She's streaming a movie again, oh man! I wish I could be watching a movie right now. I call out, "Elizabeth Campos." In the room, a lady begins to gather her stuff as she stands up. She is carrying a purse, two plastic bags full of stuff, a cane, and an umbrella. I do not remember rain in the forecast for today, and why do people almost always have to bring so much stuff with them to have blood drawn? I guess I will never know. I smile at her as I point towards the draw station. "Good morning, this way please," I say.

As I walk into the draw station after her, she sits down and looks at me and says, "You look too young, I hope you know what you're doing because I am very difficult to have my blood drawn!"

I smile at her and reply, "As a matter of fact, I do. Where did they draw your blood from the last time you had blood drawn?"

She looks at me and shrugs as she raises both of her arm sleeves. Great! Just what I need—a difficult draw when I need to draw so much blood from her. And why do older people always have to mistrust the young as being incompetent? I mean on one hand I get it: since we're young, it's unlikely we have much experience on the job and probably haven't dealt with a lot of difficult scenarios. But asking if we're any good will only make us more nervous or intimidated, and that's not going to help either one of us. I have been asked that question many times before, and depending on how nice the patient is, I sometimes tell them that I am new and this is my first day. But not this time. I already have two things on my mind that are concerning me—the fact that she needs so many tests done and the fact that she claims to be a difficult draw—and I do not want to make things worse by playing smart.

I put my gloves on as I eyeball both of her arms from the distance, and sure enough, I cannot see any veins on her. I still have to palpate them of course, but as of now, it seems like she might indeed be a difficult draw. I apply the tourniquet and begin palpating her left arm, which is resting on the table and is closer to me, and, because I have been forewarned about it, I decide to take longer and focus a lot as I feel for her veins. I feel nothing! I tell her, "I can't feel anything here so far, let me see your other arm." I switch the tourniquet to her other arm, and again I feel nothing!

Next thing I usually do when this happens is to start looking at the patient's hands and see if they have any good veins there. I try to avoid drawing blood from the hands because it usually is more painful and requires a little bit more time. Still, I tie the tourniquet on one of her wrists and then the other, looking for veins on her hands, and again there is nothing! Mrs. Campos looks at me and says, "Told you so." I smile at her in response, trying not to look worried. Lies! Inside of me I am beginning to get a little stressed out, because it already took me a while to lookup her tests on the test menu, it has already taken a while to look for a usable vein, and now it is going to take longer as I am about to pull some aces from my sleeve to try and make her veins pop up a little. All of this time it's taking is causing more work to accumulate for me as patients keep coming in. I do not want to have patients waiting for a long time, but it seems like that is what's going to happen.

I stand up and say, "Okay, Mrs. Campos, we are going to have to try some tricks in order to make your veins wake up, as they seem to be asleep this morning." She smiles. I then grab a glove and begin filling it up with warm water from the faucet, and as I am doing so I ask her, "Did you drink any water today?"

"No," she replies.

"What about yesterday, did you have a good amount of water intake?"

"No, the doctor told me to be fasting, so I have not drunk or eaten anything since about 9:00 p.m."

This happens almost every time—patients believe that fasting means not eating or drinking anything. However, water is always okay, and as a matter of fact, drinking a lot of water is great before having blood drawn because it ensures that we are hydrated, and that helps our veins be a little bit more visible. I always like to think of it as a car: if you do not put fluids in your car, it's not going to run! The body isn't much different in that sense.

I answer her, "Mrs. Campos, water is always okay, you should drink a good amount of water before going to have your blood drawn. Having enough water in you helps your veins be more visible for us. Especially since you know you are difficult to have your blood drawn, you should drink plenty of water the day before." I turn toward the office. "Deborah, could you please get some warm water for Mrs. Campos?" I yell loud enough for Deborah to hear me over the noise of the movie she is watching. Warm water is better than cold water at encouraging circulation, which in turn helps the veins become engorged.

As Deborah is bringing her a cup full of water, I tie a knot on the glove full of warm water and bring it over to the patient. I then tell her, "Mrs. Campos, please drink that water. I am also going to put this glove with warm water on your left arm. Your veins become easier for us to see if you are warm, and I could feel you are really cold right now, so please leave it there and I will be back in five minutes." She nods and drinks the water as I proactively grab the next patient's lab order and begin to make sure everything is in order and gather the needed supplies. This way, as soon as I'm done with Mrs. Campos I can just call the next patient without losing any more time. I do this for the next two patients' lab orders before the five minutes are up. Time to rock and roll now.

I walk back to the draw station and ask Mrs. Campos as I put gloves on, "It's the moment of truth, are you ready?"

"I hope so," she replies in a skeptical way. I take the glove full of water away from her arm, tie the tourniquet, and begin to feel again for a vein. Bingo! I can feel one—it is rather a small one, and it is deep in her arm so I will tie a second tourniquet on top of the first one, which I hope will help even more. People always say two are better than one, and that usually also applies in cases like this one . . . or at least I hope it does!

"Sorry, Mrs. Campos," I say. "I can feel a vein, but I need to make it look bigger, so I'm going to tie a second tourniquet around your arm. This is going to hurt a little." As soon as I tie the second tourniquet, I feel again and the vein feels much better this time. I smile, a smile of victory! I proceed to draw her blood. It takes a while for me to finish filling up all of the tubes she needs, and every time I switch a tube full of blood for an empty one, I pray in my mind that her vein continues to give enough blood to fill up the next tube. Luckily it does, and I finish drawing all of the tubes needed and labeling them before the patient leaves.

Mrs. Campos stands up from the chair she has been sitting in for the past 20 minutes and says, "Thank you, I will see you next week." I wave bye at her, smiling. Inside of me I do not know if I should be happy that she is coming back next week because she liked how I helped her, or if I should be worried that I will have to go through this again. I guess it will become easier next time as I will not be getting into unknown waters. I just hope she remembers to drink water next time!

I put away all of her labeled tubes full of blood in the tubes holder, write down the needed information on her lab order, and pick up the supplies I previously readied-up for the next patient. I take a deep breath and begin walking toward the reception area to call in the next patient. When I get there, Deborah is looking at me with a sympathetic smile, and I say, "Man, that was a tough one." She smiles and nods back at me. I better hurry, because I've got some catch-up to do if I want to go to lunch on time.

Chapter Five

Catch-Up Time

"Thank you for coming, Mr. Diaz," I say as I see the last patient of the morning rush leave. He was slightly upset because he had to wait quite a while due to Mrs. Campos' sleepy veins. Luckily I was able to talk to him and calm him down. I have now finished drawing blood on nearly 20 patients this morning. I look at the clock on the wall and it is 11:15 a.m. Where did time go? I have 45 minutes to catch up on things if I want to go to lunch at my usual time—noon—which I should be able to do as long as no more patients arrive before then.

I need to put all of the tubes of blood and the urine into specimen bags—small plastic bags that contain the lab order and the specimens for a single patient—so they can be picked up by the outside laboratory. But first I need to do some processing on them. For example, some tubes need to be spun in the centrifuge machine, and others need to be refrigerated or frozen. All the urine needs to be transferred into small tubes as well. Almost every single patient needs blood drawn in a tiger-top tube because many common tests can be tested out of the serum that is obtained once I centrifuge it. In order to centrifuge those tubes, I need to wait at least 15 minutes for the blood to clot after I collect the sample from the patient; otherwise the outside laboratory might not be able to test it, as doing so can damage their expensive testing machines.

While I normally try to be constantly spinning the tubes as soon as they sit in the tubes holder for the minimum amount required, that is almost impossible to do on Mondays because I have so many patients. This causes me to have to play catch-up as soon as the patients leave. The centrifuge can only spin eight tubes per cycle, and each cycle takes about 10 minutes. With exception of the tubes from Mrs. Campos, which I had to spin, transfer to special tubes, and refrigerate right away, I have not been able to spin any other tubes so far today. So now I grab the first eight tubes, put them in the centrifuge machine, and move on to work on the urine samples while they are spinning.

Processing urine samples is faster than processing blood tubes because there is no waiting period before I can start working on them. There are two common urine tests that require processing. One of them, which is by far the most common, is called a urinalysis with a dipstick, which tests for chemical constituents in the urine such as glucose, blood, and protein, among others.

Today I have a lot of urine samples to process, so I grab some plastic tubes with unattached yellow caps and bring them to the plate with the urine containers. These plastic tubes are what we use to process the dipsticks. Unlike the tubes I use to collect blood directly from the patients, the tubes for urine samples don't come with the cap attached to them because they don't need to be sealed with vacuum inside them (the vacuum is what sucks the blood from the patient's veins into the tubes). To fill up these dipstick tubes with the needed urine, I use a plastic pipette—a long, slender tube with a bulb on one end that can remove or dispense the desired liquid.

I open Mrs. Hernandez's urine container, squeeze the bulb on the pipette, insert it into the cup, and release the compression of the bulb so the urine is sucked into the pipette for easy transfer to the dipstick tube. Then I squeeze the appropriate amount of urine from the pipette into the dipstick tube. Lastly, I close the dipstick tube with the yellow cap, write down the patient's identifying information on the dipstick just like I do for any other tube, and place it in the plastic specimen bag that will include all specimens pertaining to Mrs. Hernandez.

The second most common urine test is a urine culture, which will test for bacteria in the urine. Processing this test requires me to transfer some of the urine from the urine container to a small tube similar to the ones for collecting blood. To do this, I use a transfer device similar to a vacutainer hub. It gets inserted into the urine cup, and it'll automatically suck up the urine into the tube, a process similar to what happens when collecting blood from the patient's arm. Once the tube is full with urine, I remove the tube from the vacutainer hub, invert it a few times so the urine gets mixed with the powdered chemical inside of it, discard the transfer device in the sharps container, label the tube with the patient's information, and then put the tube inside the specimen plastic bag.

This transfer process is usually faster and simpler than processing a dipstick, but still, it takes a bit of time as I have to be careful to not have any spills. Nobody wants to clean a urine spill or have urine splash on their clothes, right? At least not me. Luckily, I don't have any urine cultures to process today.

I have finished processing some urine samples when I hear that the centrifuge machine has come to a stop, so I unlock the lid and take out the tubes. While I take each of the tubes out, I make sure that the serum on each tube looks yellowish or pale and not red. If the serum looks red it means that it has hemolyzed—red blood cells have broken down and are mixed in the serum, when they shouldn't be there. If that happens, which could be due to an error on my part when collecting the blood or because something is happening inside of the patient's body, the outside laboratory might not be able to process the sample, and the patient might need to be called to have their blood drawn again. A hemolyzed sample can give false-positive results, among other things that are beyond my paygrade and level of training to understand, but most commonly it can cause the potassium levels to be falsely elevated on the test results. High potassium levels are very dangerous and could eventually lead a person's heart to stop, which is why it is very important that I make sure the sample was not hemolyzed due to an error on my side, such as leaving the tourniquet on for a long time or using a really small needle to draw the blood.

I check all eight tubes that were in the centrifuge, and none of them look hemolyzed—perfect! I put them apart and put the next set of eight to spin. As I do so, I hear chatting in the reception area. "Just sign in and have a seat please," I hear Deborah say. I look at my watch and it is 11:45 a.m., wow! I have only 15 minutes to help out this next patient if I want to go to lunch on time. I better get to it now. I am starting to get hungry and beginning to think of the sandwiches I have in the refrigerator.

Chapter Six

Lunch

As that patient leaves, I walk over to the reception area and see that no other patients have arrived. The clock on the wall says it is 11:58 a.m. Perfect timing—I will go on lunch now. "Can you hold the fort for a bit?" I ask Deborah.

"Sure thing," she responds, and gets back to watching her movie.

I walk over our tiny refrigerator and pull out the sandwiches, yogurt, and snacks I brought for lunch today. I would usually drive to nearby restaurants for lunch, but the city is doing some fixing on the streets, and the traffic at this time of the day becomes chaotic because lots of people are going out to lunch. So instead, I am bringing my own lunch from home, at least while the city finishes its work. I grab my lunch and head over to one of the empty rooms in the office to eat. Lately, as I go on break, I stay in the reception area and join Deborah while watching a movie, but Mondays are known for patients continuing to come in even during lunch time, so I try not to stay in patients' sight in order to not portray a bad image to them.

Today, however, I will just eat quickly and get back to catching up on the processing of the specimens. Although I am technically still on lunch and do not get paid for working during my lunch, I don't like to run behind and let work accumulate on me. If I don't get up to speed with the processing of the specimens, then later on today I'm going to run even more behind, and I might need to have patients wait for a bit as I scramble to process specimens between patients.

As I open my yogurt and begin eating, I think about how I miss my friend Roberto on days like this. He volunteered here with me for a couple of months and used to help me not fall behind with things whenever I went to lunch. We met one or two years ago at a medical terminology class, and we both decided afterwards to pursue phlebotomy education, though we went to different schools. Unfortunately for him, the place he was applying for work wanted him to have some on-the-job experience besides the time spent during his clinical internship at school. So I asked my employer if he could volunteer here, and she said it was fine for him to come and help out. It was a win-win-win situation for all three of us: I got more help, he got the experience he needed, and my employer got free labor. Fortunately for Roberto, he ended up getting the job he wanted at the hospital once he gained the experience they wanted. It was a sad time when he told me he would have to stop coming to help, but at the same time, I was happy that he could finally begin his own journey as a phlebotomist.

Once I come out of the empty room and throw away my trash, I wash my hands and begin walking toward the drawing station. As I do, I see that there are two lab orders already on the wall-mounted file holder. The two patients will have to wait for me until my lunch ends. I put gloves on and head over to the full tubes holder. By now it has been more than 15 minutes that all tiger-top tubes have been allowed to sit, so I can go straight into spinning them. I grab the next set of eight tubes and put them inside the centrifuge. I continue to transfer the urine samples from the urine containers to their respective tubes, then grab a couple of urine containers and take them to the toilet to discard the remaining urine—a not-so-fun process, but it is what I signed up for. Someone's got to do it, and it is just a small downside in the profession that you eventually become familiar with and do not really mind.

I continue spinning tubes and processing urine samples until the end of my lunch time. Then, right before my lunch break ends, I start getting everything ready to call in the two patients who have been waiting.

Chapter Seven

Kids Rush

Patients continue to come and go, but at a slower and less consistent pace compared with the morning rush. I keep processing specimens as soon as patients leave because I want to be caught up before the kids rush, which is what I call the time in the afternoon when parents tend to bring in their kids.

I never know what I will be getting once I call a kid to the draw station. It could be a baby, a toddler, a school-age kid, or a teenager. Out of all of the ages, toddlers and school-age kids are often the most challenging, not necessarily because they have small veins like babies or are a hard draw, but because their fear of pain makes them throw a tantrum as soon as they hear me calling their name.

As soon as I hear Deborah talking to someone, I make my way to the reception area and grab the lab order from her. Just by looking at the color on the lab order—red in this case—I instantly know I am dealing with a child. There's a pediatrics doctor nearby that always sends their patients to me. The laboratory that doctor's office uses always sends a red lab order. As I am making my way to the draw station to get everything ready for this draw, I am already having some peace of mind that this particular child is going to be a cooperative one. I can sense that because I don't hear any screaming or crying coming from the waiting room.

I get to the draw station and check the administrative part first as usual. Name: Dylan Robles, 2/3/2009. ICD codes are present, and insurance information is there. "A seven-year-old, shouldn't be too bad," I say to myself. I then check the tests ordered for him, but based on his age and the doctor's office he's coming from, I have a good feeling for what tests have been ordered. And when I check, I see that I was right: they ordered a CBC, lead levels, and a urine dipstick. I grab all my routine supplies as well as one lavender-top tube and make my way to call him in.

I open the door and call his name, and a young, curly-haired kid looks my way with a little bit of fright in his eyes. I try to help him overcome that from the beginning by inviting him in with a soft-voice: "Come on in, buddy." He and his mother follow me to the draw station. She sits down with the little fella on her lap.

As I'm putting my gloves on, I start making conversation with Dylan by asking him, "So, buddy, do you know why you are here today?"

He responds, "Mom said I'd be getting a little poke to see how healthy I am."

I smile at his response and reply, "As a matter of fact, you're right. I will give a little poke, and I'm not gonna lie, it will sting a little bit, but it'll be over soon as long as you don't move your arm when you feel the poke." I move my arm sideways as an example and add, "See, if you move your arm like that, or even a little bit, I might have to poke you a second time, and we don't want that, right?"

He shakes his head and says, "No."

"Exactly," I say. "And here's the deal, if you don't move, I'll give you a lollipop at the end. How would you like that?"

As he smiles at the thought of getting a lollipop, I ask him to let me see his arm, and he stretches it and lets it rest on the table. Awesome! I have his trust! This is going to go well, I say to myself.

Regardless of whether the kids were forewarned about what to expect and how to behave while at the laboratory, I always present myself to them in the most friendly and helpful way I can. There are some tricks I can use to distract them or to get them to behave better for a reward at the end. What kid does not like getting a reward or a prize?

By the way, parents play a very important role in preparing their children before they even bring them to the laboratory and also while at the draw station. Some parents, especially the ones who are not first-timers and have had other children in the past, are very knowledgeable about how to prepare their kids at home and how to help calm them down while at the laboratory. Parents with previous experience often talk to their children at home and let them know that they will be going to the laboratory to have their labs drawn, and they explain to them what to expect from the visit, including that they will feel a small pinch just like when they receive a vaccine, and that they have to stay very still until told otherwise. In my opinion, from having witnessed multiple parenting approaches to this, this is the best way to prepare children for a successful visit to the laboratory.

That was exactly the case with little Dylan today, as I see him leave happy with his well-earned lollipop. I realize what a smart young boy that was, and that he was clearly prepared well by his parents at home. While he still had some fears about what would happen, a little soft-talk from my end is often all it takes to help close that gap and calm his nerves. It gives me joy being able to help kids in a way that will not cause any additional mental trauma or increase their fears of doctor's offices or needles.

On the other hand, some other parents, especially the ones who are first-timers, do not talk to their children in advance, and just bring them to the laboratory hoping for the best. I suppose they're hoping for me to do some magic without their help. Sometimes it works, and with some last-minute good coaching from me and their parents, we might be able to get them to cooperate so I can draw their blood. Of course, the younger the kid, the more challenging it becomes to try and get them to cooperate and understand what is happening.

The worst that can happen is when parents try to teach their children a lesson, or get them to behave better at home, by threatening them with taking them to the doctor for an injection or vaccine. Doing so makes the kid associate misbehaving with getting a shot, and that only causes the kid to panic, cry, and not cooperate, because they think that they are at the laboratory to receive the punishment that their parents have been threatening. This is a no-no, parents!

For school-age kids and teenagers, I have pasted some black-and-white pictures on the cabinet doors by where the children sit to have their blood drawn. These can sometimes do the job of distracting a nervous kid. And it looks like I'm going to get the chance to test that now, because my next patient is a 10-year-old girl who I can tell right away is not happy to be here. I call her back, and she's very reluctant to get up and only does so when her mom practically drags her by the wrist. I have her sit in the seat, and I go through my speech about how she'll feel a small sting and she has to be still, and then I point to one of the pictures on the cabinet—a drawing of some treetops with several koalas hiding in the trees.

"Do you see that picture, Juana?" I ask. She nods, and I say, "Can you see there are some koalas hiding in those trees?"

"Yes, I see them," she says quietly.

"Right!" I say. "There's a lot of them hiding in those trees. I want you to count all of them, okay? If you get the number right, I have a lollipop and some stickers for you. But let me warn you, almost nobody finds them all—do you think you could do it?"

Juana nods again, and I can see just a bit of her nerves fade away as she focuses in on the picture. Her shoulders loosen just a little, and her previously tight mouth opens a tiny bit as she starts counting. By now I've already cleaned her arm with alcohol pads, and I slip the needle in. She winces, but she keeps counting animals. Before she knows it, I'm done.

"How many did you count?" I ask as I tape the bandage on.

"Eleven," she answers.

"Good job, you actually found all of them, you're so smart!" I tell her. As she and her mom head out, I give her a lollipop and let her pick a couple stickers from a cardboard box. "Thank you for being so brave and so still, Juana," I say. She gives me a big, relieved smile on the way out.

Unfortunately, that trick does not help with all kids. For some, their fear is too great to be overcome by promising them a prize. Sometimes I have the parents sit down with their kids on their laps, which can give some kids enough confidence to let me draw their blood. Other times it's not enough, and I need to get the parents to hold down the child. I have the parent put their kid's legs in between their own legs and squeeze, preventing the kid from kicking me or trying to slide away from the chair. At the same time, the parent helps me hold down the straightened arm of the kid while it rests against the table for stability. Most of the time just the strength of one parent is enough to immobilize the child this way, but oftentimes I need to ask the second parent, if present, or Deborah to help me hold down the kid's arm. Kids and even babies can display a great amount of strength when they are under a perceived threat, and this can make it very dangerous for me to proceed with the blood draw, because if they happen to get loose from their parent's grip, I could injure the kid, further antagonizing any next attempt at drawing the kid's blood.

Kids can bring a lot of joy to the laboratory with their energy and interesting conversations. Or they can make a difficult day even worse by screaming, kicking, biting, and sometimes spitting at me while I attempt to draw their blood.

Fortunately for me, today brings none of those more difficult situations, although I helped eight kids this afternoon in between adult patients. They were all very cooperative, and the ones that were a little afraid, like Juana, were welcoming enough of my pep talk that I was able to calm them down after a little bit. The lollipops and stickers proved very helpful as always. I better make sure not to run out of them for my own good.

Chapter Eight

Paperwork

As 4:00 p.m. draws closer my primary focus is to finish spinning tubes. The machine is kind of loud, and when it stops I know it's time to hustle over and replace the set of tubes with the next set. It's still quiet in the waiting room, so after making that switch I go back to the desk and begin to take care of the billing. I grab the log-in sheets and sit at the desk next to Deborah's in the reception area. The first lab order is for today's first patient, sweet Mrs. Hernandez. I write her name and date of birth, and then list all of the abbreviated tests I collected for her.

Each of the four outside laboratories we are contracted with has a separate log-in sheet, and we have to send the invoice along with the proof separately to each outside laboratory. Once I log in all of the information, I have to attach a copy of the lab order as the proof along with the log-in sheet, and then store it for my employer to do the billing at the end of the month. It's going to take me a while to get through all of these, so I better hurry!

Since this is a privately owned laboratory draw station, we do not store any patient information on our computer system, which is why I have to do the billing by handwriting everything myself. Those outside laboratories do store patients' information on their computers, so their phlebotomy employees don't have to do any handwriting themselves for billing purposes—they have a billing department that can pull that information.

I continue to write down the information for the patients seen during the day, making sure not to omit any information and that every patient is logged into their respective sheets according to the outside laboratory they belong to. After logging in about five or six more patients after Mrs. Hernandez, I hear that the centrifuge has come to a stop again, and I immediately stand up and put the next set of tubes to spin. A lot of times, depending how far behind I'm running on processing, or if I look too stressed out by the end of the day, Deborah volunteers to help out by logging the information, restocking lab supplies, or helping with other simple tasks as needed. But as of now, she is just staying put. I guess I'm not looking too overwhelmed.

The next patient to log in is Mrs. Campos. I have been pushing her form almost until the end because there are so many tests to write down, including the "weird tests" that have long names and are not easy to abbreviate. I will do us both a favor, you and me, and omit listing all of the tests she had done, but let me tell you that the more than 15 tests collected from her take a significant amount of time to write down, as well as almost a quarter of the entire log-in sheet.

I hear the centrifuge come to a stop again, and I head over to do the swap. As I do, Deborah calls out, "I got this," and takes over the logging for me at the desk. I am happy that there have been no new patients since 4:00 p.m., and with Deborah working on the billing logs, I can finish processing urine samples. After that, we'll almost be ready to call it a day. Finally, so close to going home! Woo-hoo!

Chapter Nine

End of Shift

The moment Deborah finishes up with the billing logs, she puts away all the log-in sheets and yells at me from the reception area: "What else do you need help with? I'm done over here." She knows it is time to get ready to close and go home. As usual, I ask her to restock lab supplies. In the meantime, I have finished processing the urine samples and begin my final check of everything that was done today, ensuring that all specimen processing was done correctly.

To do so, I have found that the best method is to go over each and every one of the bagged specimens we have so far. I make my way to the draw station and begin going over all of the bags, which are situated in small plastic baskets to the right of the centrifuge machine. I open the bags, take a second look at all of the tests ordered, then make sure that the tubes of blood I drew for each patient are in the correct bag. Due to the pressure that I am usually under during the day, it's just normal that I might make a mistake when bagging the specimens as I try to do it fast. Now that I have Deborah helping me stock and clean up, I can pay a lot of attention to each patient's lab order and fix any misplaced specimens.

The best way to start doing this is of course by going back to the beginning of the day. So I open the specimen bag that has the lab order and the specimens for Mrs. Maria Hernandez. I pull out the lab order and verify the ordered tests for her: a CMP, LP, CBC, HgbA1c, and UA complete. I then check the kind of tubes that are in the bag. There should be one tiger-top tube, one lavender tube, and a urine dipstick. I look in the bag, confirm that all of those tubes are indeed in the bag and that they all belong to Mrs. Hernandez, and then I close the bag by sealing it with its Ziploc-like seal.

I do not only need to ensure that the proper specimens are in the correct bag. I also need to ensure that any additional processing that was needed was performed. For example, in the case of Mrs. Elizabeth Campos, some of the tests required me to transfer the serum or plasma to a different tube, and her test for ANA needed to be refrigerated. During this last check-up, I make sure that those things were taken care of, and thankfully as I'm going through her specimen bag, I find no errors.

In the case of specimens that need to be refrigerated or frozen, due to the critical timing for processing of those tests, I almost never forget to place them at the correct temperature as soon as I collect them. I just need to make sure I don't forget to take them out of the refrigerator or the freezer at the end of the day, so I go to our specimen refrigerator and grab all of the specimen bags that I have placed inside. There are five bags in the refrigerator and only one in the freezer. To make it easier for me and everyone to identify those bags with sensitive temperature requirements, I add a big fluorescent sticker to the outside of the bags that reads either "frozen" or "refrigerated." Once I take them out of the refrigerator, I place them in the specimen box—a metal box outside of our laboratory where the outside laboratory personnel can come and pick them up.

While Deborah sweeps and mops the office, I take out the trash. When I come back in, I see that Deborah is already beginning to take away all of the remaining specimen bags from today and placing them in the specimen boxes. Sweet! I look at my watch and it is 4:55 p.m. I head inside and lock the waiting room door, because even if a patient walks in right now, I would be unable to help them and they would have to come back tomorrow.

Back inside the laboratory, I put my hoodie on and wait for Deborah to gather her stuff.

"Good night, Deborah, thank you for your help today, see you tomorrow," I say to her.

She smiles back at me, and then we leave the office together. I lock the door and walk Deborah to her car, as it's dark outside and I want to make sure she makes it to her car safely.

53

I begin making my way to my car in the dark, happy to have my hoodie because it's chilly out. I feel satisfied that I have successfully finished another day at work. Although I feel tired from the long hours, I wouldn't change anything in my job. Just like lots of people have said in the past, "Find a job that you enjoy doing, and you will never have to work a day in your life." That is exactly how I feel every day. I feel like I've not come to work, but rather just come to the laboratory and had a nice time while helping others. This feeling is particularly meaningful when I know that patients leave the lab with a better taste in their mouths.

I get in my car and get ready to drive in our dark and congested freeways. I turn up the music before I pull out of the parking lot. This is the time when I get to think about how today went. I feel especially good that I was able to help Mrs. Campos regardless of how challenging it was to draw her blood and get all of her tests ready for testing. She didn't only leave happy that I didn't have to poke her multiple times, she left willing to come back and be helped again by someone who she at first distrusted. Also, I smile at the memory of how smart and well-prepared little Dylan was for his blood draw today.

As I get closer to home, I think about how I will spend the rest of the evening, but part of my mind is also looking ahead to the challenges and satisfactions that tomorrow has in store for me. Whatever they are, I'm satisfied and thankful that I'm able to help others. Life is good, let us hope it stays that way for a long time.

About the Author

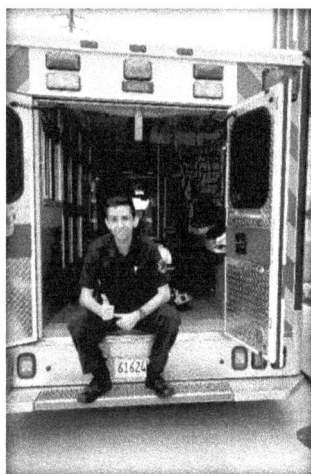

Jonathan I. Angulo became a licensed phlebotomist at the age of 20. From there, his passion for the medical field and for helping other people has led him to pursue other careers in healthcare, most recently becoming a paramedic during the Covid-19 pandemic. He has devoted his life to helping people in need and currently volunteers at a free clinic for low-income people at his local church by serving as a board member. When he is not at work, Jonathan enjoys walking, reading, and practicing archery. Jonathan currently works from home, as he, heartbreakingly, had to stop providing direct care to patients while battling cancer. He eagerly hopes to defeat his disease soon so he can go back to caring for patients and continue his education in pursuit of becoming a nurse practitioner.

LEARN TO USE
A QR CODE

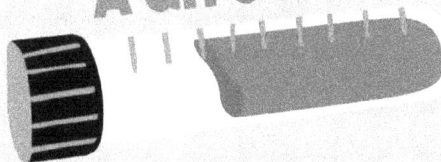

1 Open your camera and point your device at the QR code

2 Wait for camera to recognize and scan QR code

3 Click banner or notification when it appears on your screen

OKAY

4 Information associated with the QR code will automatically load

Note: Older phones might require that you download a QR scanner app first.

Stay informed about upcoming books and learn more.

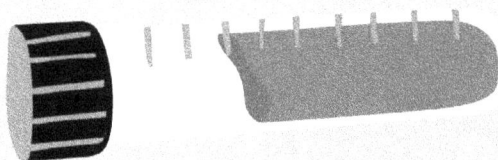

Coming Soon:

- **A DAY IN THE LIFE OF A PHLEBOTOMIST**

  - Hospital Edition

VISIT THE AUTHOR'S WEBSITE
anguloauthor.com

Sign up for announcements and discounts

Explore other books

Contact the author

LEARN HOW TO BECOME A PHLEBOTOMIST AND BEGIN YOUR OWN JOURNEY

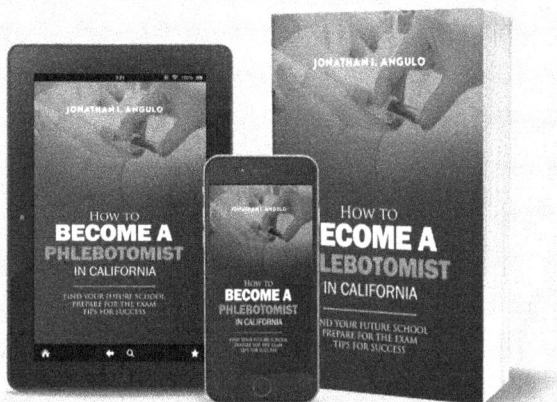

Let a professional phlebotomist guide you, step-by-step, on how to navigate the process of becoming a phlebotomist.

TAKE YOUR FUTURE IN YOUR OWN HANDS.

Read on to look at Chapter One!

JONATHAN I. ANGULO

How To
BECOME A
PHLEBOTOMIST
IN CALIFORNIA

FIND YOUR FUTURE SCHOOL
PREPARE FOR THE EXAM
TIPS FOR SUCCESS

Chapter One

Why Become a Phlebotomist?

Phlebotomy is a very important and rewarding profession in the healthcare field. It is not for nothing that phlebotomists are often called the backbone of the hospital or laboratory.

Phlebotomists are healthcare professionals who assist in the running of laboratories mainly by collecting blood specimens. They help process most of the specimens collected as well as any that are brought to the laboratory, ensuring they are ready to be tested right away or to be sent to an outside laboratory. Their most valuable skill is the ability to collect blood samples from patients of all ages. Believe it or not, it is because of this valuable and perfected-over-time skill that even nurses and doctors go looking for phlebotomists to help them with difficult draws. (Fun fact: we call patients a "difficult draw" if it is not so easy to draw their blood right away, and they require multiple attempts; there are many reasons why this might happen.)

However, phlebotomists also help with collecting and handling other samples, such as sputum, urine, and stool. More recently, they have also stepped up to the call and provided enormous help in the collection of swabs for Covid testing and even given vaccines.

There are five main reasons why you might want to become a phlebotomist:

1. Accessible New Career

Training to become a phlebotomist is a relatively easy way to become a healthcare professional and join the medical field. It takes only 80–100 hours of training to become eligible to apply for licensure in California. It is also not too expensive— you can easily complete your schooling for less than $2,000. Compare that with other entry-level careers, such as becoming a medical assistant, for example. They go to go school for about nine months to a year and can spend more than $10,000. The lower cost and shorter training period do not only provide an easier road to launching your career. They are also a lower price to pay to find out if working in the medical field is what you want to pursue after all. I don't know about you, but in my own case, my wallet would be much happier if I found out that the medical field is not for me before committing to longer and more expensive training.

2. Opportunity to Work at a Job that Matters

Collecting blood and other specimens is of utmost importance in the care of a patient. The most common procedure you will become proficient at will be collecting blood samples via what is called a venipuncture, or the puncture of a vein. With the samples you draw, doctors are able to determine if a patient needs a new medication or if their current medication is helping the way it is expected to. They can find out if someone has a disease and what they can do to treat it, they can find out if someone needs a blood transfusion, and many other things. The phlebotomist is the lynchpin to all that information.

3. Multiple Job Locations

Remember the day you had blood drawn at your doctor's office? Or the time you went to a laboratory (such as Quest Diagnostics, LabCorp, or ABC laboratories, to name a few) to have blood drawn? How about the time you or a family member were at a hospital, and someone came to your bedside to collect blood? It is highly likely that the person who collected the sample was a phlebotomist. That is one of the perks of being a phlebotomist—there are lots of places at which you could be hired. Here are some common work places and job titles.

Work Places
Doctor's Offices
Private Laboratories
Urgent Cares
Hospitals
Mobile Phlebotomists
Blood Donation Centers
Dialysis Centers
Covid-19 Collection Sites

Job Titles
Phlebotomist
CPT-1
Laboratory Technician
Lab Assistant
Travel Phlebotomist
Specimen Processor

Different work places might give their employees different job titles and different responsibilities, but becoming a phlebotomist opens the door for you to be hired at all these places and perform a variety of duties specific to each work place.

4. Good Pay for the Level of Experience
So, what is the pay like? Well, it depends on your experience, the type of place where you are hired, whether you are a full-time or part-time employee, and perhaps your ability to negotiate your pay rate. As of May 2021, according to the U.S. Bureau of Labor Statistics, California is the state with both the highest annual mean wage, at $48,070, and highest hourly mean wage, at $23.11. Not too bad, right? Of course, nothing is set in stone, and you could find yourself making more than that in no time.

5. Growing Job Market
On another good note from the U.S. Bureau of Labor Statistics, California is the state with the highest employment level for phlebotomists. Also, the employment rate for phlebotomists at the national level is projected to grow 22 percent between 2020 and 2030, a rate that is

significantly higher than the average of 8 percent for all other occupations. This is great news for a future phlebotomist! You are going to be joining a profession that is projected to grow significantly in the coming years. That means more job openings and more opportunities for you to succeed.

In the next chapter, you'll find some often overlooked but important tips to address before you begin your phlebotomy classes.

www.ingramcontent.com/pod-product-compliance
Lightning Source LLC
Chambersburg PA
CBHW050601280326
41933CB00011B/1940